T0196352

The

little

Red Book

The

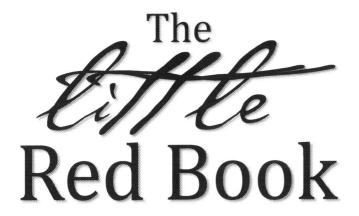

Red Book

A "Bedroom Talk" Dictionary

Includes sexy phrases, erotic bedtime short stories,
and a fun "Sex To-Do List" fill-in sheet
for fulfilling fantasies.

ANN MARIE RIOS

iUniverse LLC
Bloomington

The Little Red Book
A "Bedroom Talk" Dictionary

iUniverse books may be ordered through booksellers or by contacting:

iUniverse LLC
1663 Liberty Drive
Bloomington, IN 47403
www.iuniverse.com
1-800-Authors (1-800-288-4677)

ISBN: 978-1-4759-9481-0 (sc)
ISBN: 978-1-4759-9482-7 (hc)
ISBN: 978-1-4759-9483-4 (ebk)

Library of Congress Control Number: 2013910828

Printed in the United States of America

iUniverse rev. date: 07/18/2013

"Living in a world where texts and tweets rule and communication is always evolving, The Little Red Book offers a refreshingly fun and sexy look into improving sexual communication within relationships. Ann Marie Rios strives to enhance our ability for creative imagination and sexual fantasy, while igniting the dirty talker within us all for more exciting, passionate, and pleasurable sex lives."

Dr. Hernando Chaves M.F.T., D.H.S.
Licensed CA Marriage and Family Therapist, Doctor of Human Sexuality, Clinical Sexologist, Human Sexuality Professor.

The Little Red Book is a welcoming, informative, and fun guide, providing couples with just enough support and inspiration to do their own exploring.

Chauntelle Anne Tibbals, Ph.D. - Sociologist

This book is dedicated to all couples—in new or in finely aged relationships—that want to reignite a spark or help keep their fire burning.

This book is also dedicated to all the hopeful singles out there that want to be ready when the time, and right person, comes along.

Contents

Preface

This book has been many years in the making. As someone who has made a living at "bedroom talk" for the last decade, I came to discover a deeper emotional connection not only with my lover, but also with the vixen inside me. I found that a deeper emotional connection between my lover and me came through the intimate thoughts that we shared, the words we used to describe them, and the trust we developed as we have a safe, sexual arena to explore together.

As the host of a nationally broadcast radio show designed around intimate stories, sex topics, and "sexy talk" in the bedroom, I have been amazed at how many people ask me about the same issue: having trouble talking sexy in the bedroom with their lover or not being able to get their lover to talk back to them. The desire was there, but the comfort level or know-how was not yet present.

Through my life experience, research, and self-practice, I have compiled a collection of information to build a solid foundation for your intimate life.

This book is written for couples of all demographics, including new or aged relationships and hopeful singles. This book is helpful to anyone looking to improve bedroom vocabulary, adding fun to his or her bedroom behavior.

Acknowledgments

I would like to thank all the listeners of my radio show on SiriusXM who took the time to become callers into my program on Playboy Radio. This includes the many people who shared their stories, concerns, and questions on how to spice up the "bedroom talk" with their partner.

Your many calls, with similar questions and concerns, were the motivation to write this book.

Introduction

The purpose of the A–Z is to expand your sexy vocabulary and give you ideas of how to use adjectives to help develop a "bedroom dialogue."

The spotlight-on-body-parts section is to expand your vocabulary when it comes to referring to parts of your or your partner's body.

The purpose of the short stories is to show dialogue examples, and they make for great bedtime stories.

The carnal-knowledge section is simply to share some of the physical and emotional benefits of sex.

The spotlight-on-fetishes section is to introduce some sexual practices that you may not be familiar with, so that they no longer seem so foreign or intimidating to you and your partner.

The purpose of the fill-in sheets is not only for fun but to encourage you to create your own short stories.

Last but definitely not least, the "Sex To-Do List" tear-out sheet is to create a fun list of sexual adventures that you want to live out, and then going about your intimate adventure.

The goal is to help create a sexually open mind.

General Sexy Talking Tips

1. Think of the goal as seducing your lover with words.

2. Draw from your five senses: touch, taste, sound, scent, and sight.

3. When role-playing, use words that are particular to that character or that character's "job duties." When having sexual activities in new or creative places, include words and descriptions that relate to the environment you are in as well.

4. Laugh off any mistakes, and move on quickly. The purpose of this is to have fun, so don't stress. The more you practice, the more comfortable you will be, and a better talker you will quickly become.

*__Tip:__ When role-playing, search the house ahead of time for objects and props that your character will need.

Building on Your "Bedroom Vocabulary"

A-Z

A

Admire: admire

"I *admire* the way you always _____ to please me."
"Sometimes I like to just sit back and *admire* your _____."
Synonyms: appreciate, treasure, worship

adore

"One of the many things I *adore* about your bedroom behavior is the way you _____."
Synonyms: idolize

adventurous

"Why don't we see how *adventurous* we can be this summer and have sex on the beach at night under the stars, or . . . .
Synonyms: daring

amuse

"You always *amuse* me when you tickle me with a feather or when you _____."
Synonyms: charm, please

anal

"A few things we can use to slowly explore *anal* satisfaction are fingers, small-sized vibrators, and of course, the tongue."
Synonyms: butthole sex.

anchor

"I want you to drop it deep inside of me and leave it in there like an *anchor*."
"I want to drop it deep inside of you and leave it in there like an *anchor*."
Synonyms: weight

arouse

"You can always *arouse* me when you _____."
Synonyms: stimulate

ass

"You have the most amazing *ass*. I love to watch it move when I do you from behind."
"Put your hands on my *ass* and squeeze as I ride you."
Synonyms: booty, buns (See also body-parts section.)

attraction

"I have always had an *attraction* to the way you _____."
Synonyms: appeal

B

bare

"There is nothing quite as nice as our *bare* bodies next to each other." "What about soaking our *bare* bodies together in a nice, hot bubble bath?"
Synonyms: naked, nude, undressed

bliss/blissful

"I'm in such a state of *bliss* after every time we make love." "It is so *blissful* every time we try something new."
Synonyms: euphoria, paradise

blowjob

"It is always a great start to my day when you wake me up with one of your amazing *blowjobs*."
"Why don't you join me in the shower so I can give you a wet *blowjob* without thinking about how messy it might get."
Synonyms: cock sucking, fellatio, head, oral

bondage

"What do you think about trying some light *bondage*? We can take turns tying each other up with an old pair of stockings or those old ties."
Synonyms: restraint

breasts

"I love when you let me be your captain and motorboat your beautiful *bosom*."
Synonyms: boobs, bosom (See also body-parts section.)

built

"Your legs were *built* to wear stockings; they fit you so well."
"Your body was *built* for wearing _____; you look amazing in them."
Synonyms: created, made

bust

"You make me feel so good, I'm going to *bust*!"
Synonyms: erupt, explode

C

caboosing.

The act of having sex on a moving train.
"What do you think about us planning a trip by train this year, so we can join the *caboosing* club?"
Synonyms: train banging

camel toe.

The visual effect created when a woman's pants cling too tightly to the crotch, emphasizing the shape of the vaginal lips.
"It's so sexy when you wear _____, because I can see a bit of *camel toe*. It is such a turn-on."
Synonyms: moose-knuckle wedgie

captivate

"When you go down on me, the way you look up at me completely *captivates* me."
Synonyms: entrance, mesmerize

caress

"The way you *caress* me on my _____ gives me goose bumps."
Synonyms: fondle, touch

charm

"Keep doing that, and you're going to *charm* the pants right off me."
Synonyms: sweet talk

clitoris

"One of my favorite sensations is when you/I suck on my/ your *clitoris*."
Synonyms: clit

consume

"I want to kiss you all over and *consume* you."
Synonyms: devour

cream/creamy.

Additional words that can be used to describe cum or other bodily fluids.
"I can't wait to taste your *cream*-filled center."
"It's so exciting when you explode and *cream* all over me."
Synonyms: pussy juice, semen

cum

"Give me _____ seconds of a warning before you *cum*, so I can be ready and we can *cum* together."
Synonyms: climax, orgasm

D

dance/dancing.

Bouncing up and down on the cock, with enthusiasm.
"It felt amazing last night the way you were *dancing* all over my cock."
"How about we go salsa *dancing*, then later I can *dance* around on your cock?"
Synonyms: riding the cock

daring

"Next time you're in a *daring* mood, why don't we have sex in/ at _____?"
Synonyms: adventurous, bold

dazzle

"Every time you use your tongue to _____, you *dazzle* me."
Synonyms: overwhelm

deep-throat.

To perform fellatio (dick sucking) to where the penis is sticking in the throat, causing a gag reflex.
"You know just how to *deep-throat* me. I love your mouth."
"Sit back, baby. Let me see how far I can *deep-throat* you."
Synonyms: swallow

delicious

"Your body always tastes *delicious*, especially when _____"
Synonyms: delightful, pleasing

delight

"When you tell me to _____, it is pure *delight*."
Synonyms: bliss, ecstasy, pleasure

desire

"I *desire* you most when you _____."
Synonyms: fancy

discipline

"If you insist on being naughty, I'm going to have to *discipline* you, maybe with a bare-bottom spanking."
Synonyms: punish

dom/dominant

"Next time we role-play, we should take turns being the *dom* or *dominant* in our adventure."
Synonyms: authority/authoritarian

dominatrix

"What do you think about me buying you a black latex outfit, so one night you can be my *dominatrix* and I'll be your willing sex slave?"
Synonyms: mistress

E

electric

"Your kiss, your touch, your scent . . . Everything about you is *electric*."
Synonyms: dynamic, spirited

enchanting

"The way you _____ is completely *enchanting*."
Synonyms: captivating

entice

"Even when I may not be feeling in the mood, you know just how to *entice* me by _____."
Synonyms: attract, lure, tempt

erection

"You can always put me in the mood and give me an *erection* when you suck on my earlobes or my _____."
"I love feeling your *erection* grow against me through your pants."
Synonyms: boner, chubby, hard-on, stiffy

erotic

"I was thinking of buying an *erotic* storybook so we can read each other an *erotic* bedtime story at night, and then maybe make our own."
Synonyms: sensual, sensuous, sexy

excited

"I can't help but get *excited* every time you _____."
Synonyms: enthusiastic, impassioned

F

fantasy

"What *fantasy* would you like to live out next time? We should make a list . . ."
Synonyms: dream

feisty

"You are extra amazing when you get *feisty* like a firecracker."
Synonyms: fiery

fellatio

"You are utterly fantastic at *fellatio*, my dear."
Synonyms: blowjob, cock sucking, deep-throating, giving head, hummer, oral, sucking dick

fetish

"How about we try out one new *fetish* a month? We can take turns each month choosing which one, and you can go first."
Synonyms: sexual adventure

fill up

"Oh, yes, baby. I can't wait to feel you *fill* me *up*!"
"It is such an amazing treat when you tell me to *fill* you *up* with my love."
Synonyms: fulfill, internal ejaculation

flirt

"It still turns me on just as much as when we first started dating whenever you *flirt* with me."
Synonyms: tease

frisky

"I can tell you're feeling *frisky* when you _____."
Synonyms: horny

flash

"Why don't we wear nothing but trench coats next time we go grocery shopping late night, so we can *flash* each other as we pass in the aisles."
Synonyms: expose, show off

flood

A *flood* of juices as I brought her to orgasm let me know I had finally stimulated her G-spot.
Synonyms: explosion, gush

flowing

Our juices were *flowing* as we made love on the kitchen table.
Synonyms: running

fox

"You are one sexy *fox*!"
Synonyms: vixen

G

glorious

We had a *glorious* time skinny-dipping in our pool on a hot summer day.
Synonyms: enjoyable, gratifying, magnificent

glow/glowing

They were both *glowing* after sneaking away to have sex, then returning to the party.
Synonyms: blushing, flushed

gorgeous

"You were the most *gorgeous* woman at the party tonight."
Synonyms: dazzling

going up inside

"I love the feeling of *going up inside* you when we have sex standing up."
"I love the feeling of you *going up inside* me when we have sex standing up."
Synonyms: entering

grand

Eating chocolate syrup and strawberries off each other was a *grand* experience to share.
Synonyms: great

great

"Come here, baby. Let me kiss that *great,* big, gorgeous cock."
Synonyms: enormous, gigantic, huge

grateful

"I am *grateful* to you for your love and for your oral skills."
Synonyms: obliged, thankful

grope

I told him to *grope* my body in the darkness, with nothing more than candlelight.
Synonyms: feel, probe

G-spot

The best way to stimulate her *G-spot* is to insert the first two fingers, fingerprints facing upward and massage that soft button of inner tissue about two inches deep and toward the roof of the vagina. Rub the clitoris to help her relax if she begins to tighten up.
Synonyms: love button, Gräfenberg spot

gush

As he continued to stimulate my G-spot, I *gushed* all over the sheets.
Synonyms: squirted

gyrate

"When you grind and *gyrate* on me, it sends me over the edge."
Synonyms: revolve, twirl

H

handsome

"Baby, you are still as *handsome* as the day we met."
Synonyms: attractive

heart

"You make my *heart* skip a beat when you _____."
Synonyms: soul

heat

"Baby, you sure know how to bring the *heat*."
Synonyms: excitement, hotness

heated

A *heated* phone sex conversation always makes the sex spicier next time.
Synonyms: fierce, impassioned, passionate

hole

"I want you to enter my *hole* like you are a golfer aiming for a *hole*-in-one."
"I want to kiss and lick you from one sexy *hole* to another."
Synonyms: opening

hot

They were both so *hot* with excitement when they heard sounds of sex coming from the hotel room next door, that they began to have sex themselves.
Synonyms: aroused, heated, sultry

horny

"I can't help but become *horny* when you _____."
Synonyms: aroused, turned on

hug

"Let me *hug* you, because I love how close it makes me feel to you."
"Let me *hug* your cock with my lips."
Synonyms: embrace, squeeze

hunger

"When we go a few days without having sex, I begin to *hunger* for your love."
Synonyms: appetite, lust

hump

Dry *humping* can be an extreme turn-on when you are having a make-out session.
Synonyms: grinding

I

impressive

"That new move you used on me from our Kama Sutra book was *impressive*."
Synonyms: awe-inspiring, awesome

immense

The nipple clamps we tried out brought us both *immense* excitement.
Synonyms: monumental, tremendous

impulse

I got the *impulse* to join my lover in the shower this morning. How amazing that turned out to be!
Synonyms: inspiration

inhibitions

"This weekend when we go away, let's leave our *inhibitions* at home and just enjoy every moment and every new thing we try."
Synonyms: constraints, suppressions

intense

Whenever we explore tying each other up or _____, we both feel an *intense* passion.
Synonyms: passionate, strong

intimate

Taking and making the time to be *intimate* with your partner is what will help keep your sex life strong.
Synonyms: sexual

intoxicating

Making love in the rain was an *intoxicating* idea.
"Your kisses are intoxicating."
Synonyms: alluring, enticing

J

jam it in

"I love when you take control and tell me to *jam it in* you."
"It feels so good when you *jam it in* me."
Synonyms: penetrate, push, shove

jiggle

"Just lie back and let me *jiggle* on your cock."
"It drives me wild when you *jiggle* all over my cock."
Synonyms: bounce, grind

juggle

"Hold on to my breasts while I ride you, so it feels like you are trying to *juggle* them."
Synonyms: jiggle, shuffle.

juicy

"It is so sexy how *juicy* you get when I _____."
"You make me feel so *juicy* when you _____."
Synonyms: moist, succulent, wet

K

Kama Sutra.

Book that shows sexual positions and gives other helpful tips. It contains instructions and pictures of several different positions of intercourse. The goal of this book is for more variety and gratification in your sexual practices.
"I think we should try one of these Kama Sutra positions at least once a week/month. Some of them look really fun and are a twist on our favorite positions."
Synonyms: sculptural positions

kindle

Kissing by the fireplace began to *kindle* even more heat.
Synonyms: ignite

kinky

"You are so sexy when you come up with new *kinky* ideas for places to do it outside the bedroom."
Synonyms: erotic

kiss

"Let me *kiss* your body from north to south."
Synonyms: smooch

L

large

"Your cock is *large* and in charge."
Synonyms: big, enormous, gigantic, huge, massive

lick

"I am going to lick both nipples before traveling south."
She began to *lick* the tip of his dick like an ice-cream cone.
Synonyms: taste

limber

A regular practice of yoga made her body very *limber,* and she was then flexible enough to try out some of the Kama Sutra poses she had talked about with her partner.
Synonyms: flexible

linger

He *lingered* with his face between her thighs after he brought her to orgasm.
Synonyms: idled

longing

They were *longing* to be next to each other.
Synonyms: desiring, yearning

love

"I *love* the way you put your hands all over my body."
Synonyms: adore

lubricate

She began to *lubricate* his cock by putting it in her mouth before she slipped him insider her.
Synonyms: moisten

lucky

My wife told me she bought some new lingerie. I think I'm getting *lucky* in the bedroom tonight.
Synonyms: fortunate

luscious

"One of my favorite things about you is your *luscious* figure.
Synonyms: voluptuous

lust

"I have been *lusting* after you all day ever since you sent me that naughty text this morning."
Synonyms: crave, hunger, yearn

M

magnificent

My lover put on a *magnificent* striptease show for me.
Synonyms: exquisite, majestic

magnetic

"One of the things that has always drawn me to you is your *magnetic* personality."
Synonyms: captivating

man nectar

"I love to feel you fill me up with your warm *man nectar*."
Synonyms: love juice

marvelous

It's important to try new things with your partner so that you both feel like you have a *marvelous* lover.
"Baby, the way you use your ____ to ____ me is simply *marvelous*."
Synonyms: amazing, wonderful

massage

Giving your partner a happy-ending massage is a great way to show affection.
Synonyms: caress, stimulate, stroke

mesmerize

"You still *mesmerize* me every time you _____."
Synonyms: enchant

Mile High Club.

Refers to two people engaging in sexual intercourse at an altitude of no less than 5,280 feet above the earth (a "mile high") in an airplane.

Great things to bring when planning to join the Mile High Club: your own blanket, wipes for cleanup, and a great excuse for why you both need to be in the bathroom at once in case the flight is full and doing it in your seat is not an option. More easily accomplished on night flights when the cabin lights are off. Most people are sleeping, and the flight attendants walk around less.

Synonyms: mile-highers

mistress

A dominant woman who has authority or control over her submissive partner in BD/SM role-play.

"Yes, *mistress*, I love when you _____."

Synonyms: dominatrix

moan

"I know I'm doing things right when I hear you begin to *moan*."

Synonyms: squeal

moist

"You always know how to make me *moist*."

Synonyms: damp, wet

morning wood.

A morning erection that is naturally caused as the brain enters the REM sleep phase.

"I love to wake my honey up in the morning by putting my mouth all over his *morning wood.*"

"It's always a great surprise to wake up with your mouth on my *morning wood.*"

Synonyms: morning glory, pitching a tent

N

naked

"Remember that one time we saw a couple swimming in the lake *naked*? Tonight that *naked* couple should be us."
Synonyms: butt-naked, nude

ninja sex.

Sexual escapades performed in secret without any vocals or sounds. Usually done around other people, to which you are trying to remain anonymous or undetected. Can be done fully nude, but most often is done with partial clothing.
"Since we have family staying at the house over the holidays, we'll have to have *ninja sex*."
"When we go camping with our friends this summer, we can still have *ninja sex* in the tent."
Synonyms: undetected sexual encounter

nipples

"Please don't stop sucking on my *nipples*; it makes me so wet."
"It feels amazing when you rub my cock on your *nipples*."
Synonyms: areolas

nipple clamps

"If you like when I squeeze your nipples during sex, maybe we should try out some *nipple clamps* next time."
Synonyms: boob pinchers

nude

"You look great in anything you wear, but you look best when *nude*."
Synonyms: naked

nympho/nymphomaniac

"I've never enjoyed anything more than I enjoy being with you. You are turning me into a *nympho*!"
Synonyms: freak, sexaholic

O

on top

"I love all the positions we try, but there's nothing better than being *on top*."
Synonyms: cowgirl

oral

"Let's tease and please each other tonight using only our *oral* skills."
Synonyms: lingual

order

"When you *order* me to move faster, it is such a turn-on."
Synonyms: direct, instruct

orgasm

"When you use your fingers and your tongue at the same time, it brings on the most amazing *orgasm*."
Synonyms: climax

overcome

We were *overcome* with the feeling to have a quickie, so we snuck away to search for a good place to do so.
Synonyms: compelled

P

palm

An open *palm* is best when handing out sensual spankings.
Synonyms: hand

passionate

"Every time we're together is just as *passionate* as the first time."
Synonyms: emotional, excitable

please

"Tell me something new I can do to *please* you tonight."
Synonyms: pleasure

plunge

He *plunged* his hard cock into her wet pussy, and she asked him for more.
Synonyms: dip

pretty

"Sit down, my *pretty.* Let me please you tonight."
He told her what a *pretty* pussy she had before he tasted her.
Synonyms: beautiful, pleasant

provocative

"I enjoy watching you put on pantyhose, because it is very *provocative* to me."
"When you loosen your tie and look at me, it is very *provocative* and sexy."
Synonyms: stimulating, tantalizing

pull

"Next time, don't *pull* out. I want to feel you explode inside of me."
Synonyms: extract

Pulling your partner's hair is a great thing to do to intensify sex. Just make sure to grab hair near the scalp, so the *pull* feels pleasurable and not painful.
Synonyms: tug

Q

quickie

"Can you come home for lunch today? And by *lunch*, I mean a *quickie*."

Synonyms: nooner

quiver

"When you pleasure me with your mouth, it makes my whole body *quiver*."

Synonyms: quake, shiver

R

radiant

"You have the most *radiant* after-sex glow every time we make love. It is incredibly beautiful."
Synonyms: beaming

release

"Tell me when you are getting close, so we can both *release* at the same time."
Synonyms: orgasm
To *release* someone, as in BDSM play or role-play.
Synonyms: free

restraint

"You have me so worked up I am going to have to use all my self-control to *restrain* myself from finishing early."
Synonyms: self-discipline
Items such as rope or a silk scarf that you might use as a *restraint* to tie up your lover.
Synonyms: suppression

reveal

"I go wild when I watch you *reveal* your _____ to me."
Synonyms: unveil

rhythm

"Last night our bodies moved in perfect *rhythm*, and I almost could not contain myself."
Synonyms: flow

ride/rode

"She *rode* my cock all night last night and then let me finish inside her."
"He sure took me for a *ride* last night when he used that move we saw in our Kama Sutra book."
Synonyms: mount

rise

"I love kissing your cock and watching it *rise* before my eyes."
"*Rise* and shine, baby. I think we have time for a quickie."
Synonyms: arise

roadside sex

Sexual intercourse against the side of the car just before sunset or on top of the hood underneath the star-filled sky.
"Next time we're on a long road trip, let's make sure to make a pit stop for some *roadside sex!*"
Synonyms: road-edge sex

role-play

"I've always had a fantasy about a hot cop, so baby, why don't you handcuff and arrest me tonight?"
Every couple should take turns *role-playing* to safely fulfill each other's fantasies.
Synonyms: acting

romance

"I love the way you *romance* me between the sheets."
Synonyms: enchantment

romantic

"When you slip love notes into my bag, and then I find them at work, I realize how *romantic* you can be."
Synonyms: passionate

S

satisfy

"You never fail to *satisfy* me."
The long, passionate lovemaking session by candlelight *satisfied* them both.
Synonyms: exhilarate, gratify, please

sensational

"You are a *sensational* kisser, and I love when you sneak up and kiss me."
Synonyms: breathtaking, divine, incredible, mind-blowing

senses

When engaging in foreplay, work on stimulating all five of the *senses*: touch, taste, sight, smell, and sound.
Synonyms: perception

sensational

A *sensational* phone sex session while they were apart kept things spicy.
Synonyms: exciting, stimulating

sensual

The *sensual touch* of his fingertips across her back made her tingle and got her aroused.
Synonyms: passionate, stimulating

sex

She created a sexy scavenger hunt for him to find her, with *sex* to mark the spot.
Synonyms: coitus

sex up

"I want to *sex* you *up*. Let's go into the bedroom so I can put my mouth all over you."
Synonyms: copulate

The only intent of her putting on silky stockings was to *sex up* the outfit.
Synonyms: intensify

sext/sexting

A good way to keep the spark alive while away from your partner is to *sext*.
"*Sexting* with you all day long is all the foreplay I need."
Synonyms: phone sex messages

sexy

"I cannot wait until I see you in the *sexy* new piece of lingerie I bought for you."
My lover looks *sexiest* when waking up first thing in the morning, after we have made love all night long.
Synonyms: seductive

sexy time.

A fun term used to describe the lovemaking time you are planning or desiring to set aside for you and your partner. "Baby, come home early from work if you can, so we can sneak in some *sexy time* before I have to start cooking dinner for the family tonight."
Synonyms: lovemaking

sexual

When my lover and I drink wine, we are in a far more *sexual* mood.
Synonyms: erotic, passionate, sultry

shivers

Every time we touch, my body still *shivers* with anticipation of what is to come.
Synonyms: quiver, tremble

silky

"I never mind giving you a massage, because I love to touch your *silky* skin."
Synonyms: soft, tender

skinny-dipping

Every month under the full moon, my lover and I take the night to ourselves to go *skinny-dipping*."
Synonyms: nude swimming

slave.

A willing participant in submission/domination play, as a fetish or sexual stimulant.
"Starting right now, I am your willing sex *slave* for the next twenty-four hours."
Synonyms: servant, subservient

slip

"I love the way you kiss me all over before you slip your _____ inside my _____."
Synonyms: glide, insert, slide

slow

A *slow* lovemaking session is nice every once in a while.
Synonyms: leisurely

spanking.

An activity where consenting adults strike each other on the butt to induce sexual pleasure.
"I've/you've been very naughty. I think I/you deserve a *spanking*."
Synonyms: smack

spent

After a two-hour lovemaking session, we were both *spent*.
Synonyms: depleted, finished

squirt

I knew I had finally found her G-spot when she had an intense orgasm and began to *squirt* all over me.
Synonyms: eject, spray

steamy

We had a *steamy* make-out session in the car.
"Let's take a *steamy* hot shower together."
Synonyms: passionate, sexy

stiffen

When I put on my lover's favorite slow song, and dance around in my heels, I can see him start to *stiffen* in the pants. It really turns us both on.
Synonyms: harden, solidify

stimulate

I love when I wake up in the morning and the first thing I feel is my lover reaching over with finger or tongue to *stimulate* me. It makes me really wet and always puts me in the mood.
Synonyms: arouse, touch

straddle

As she began to *straddle* her lover, and kiss her way down his chest, he knew he was the one in for a ride.
Synonyms: mount, ride

strip

He put on an amazing *strip* show for her, and then he picked her up and carried her into the bedroom.
Synonyms: undress

striptease.

This is the act of taking off one's clothes and is something every couple should do for each other from time to time. Take turns between partners and incorporate different costumes/ characters to keep it exciting.
"Sit back and let me put on a *striptease* show for you with this costume you bought me."
Synonyms: strip show

stroke

"Baby, just sit back and relax and let me *stroke* your cock and make you feel good."
Synonyms: caress

stunning

"After all this time we have been together, you are still *stunning!*"
Synonyms: gorgeous, impressive, sensational, spectacular, wonderful

submit

As he looked at her in her shiny, latex corset, sexier than ever, he had no choice but to *submit* to her.
Synonyms: surrender

succulent

He buried his face between her thighs and brought them both pleasure as he enjoyed her *succulent* pussy.
Synonyms: luscious, moist, tasty

sultry

"Baby, when you look at me that way, you are so *sultry*."
Synonyms: passionate, provocative, scorching, seductive

sweetheart

Every couple should have a term such as *sweetheart* for their partner.
Synonyms: babe, baby, boo, cutie, companion, darling, dear, honey, pet name, sweetie, sugar

swing/swinger.

Couples who enjoy sexual relations outside their monogamous relationship, usually as an organized activity, like a swing party. Exchanging of spouses for sexual activities.
"What do you think about going to a *swinger* party, just to watch?"
Synonyms: sexual exchange

T

taste

We used strawberries and whipped cream to taste off each other's bodies before tasting each other.
Synonyms: savor

tempt

"Keep walking around the house naked, and you're going to tempt me to call in sick to work."
Synonyms: influence, persuade

temptation

The *temptation* to kiss him/her on the back of the neck was too much to resist.
Synonyms: allure

tender

A *tender* touch of the feather across her body was a fun new experience.
Synonyms: dainty, delicate

thirst

"I have a *thirst* for our bodies to be close together."
Synonyms: desire, longing, yearning

thrill

"The way you _____ gives me a *thrill*. Don't ever stop."
Synonyms: sensation, stimulation

throb/throbbing

His cock was *throbbing* with excitement as he watched her undress for him.
Synonyms: pulsate

tight

He tied her up with a *tight* knot. She asked him to make the ropes just a little bit tighter.
Also known as a slang term for a small vagina that is stretched out a little when it is entered. Every woman should have a *tight* pussy.
Synonyms: firm

tingle

"Your touch makes me *tingle* all over."
Synonyms: flutter, thrill

tongue

"I love when you put your *tongue* in my mouth, between my toes, or _____"
"I'm going to spell out something on your body, using my *tongue*."
Synonyms: mouth muscle

touch

"Blindfold me, then *touch* me anywhere you like."
Synonyms: caress, handle

toward the sky

"This time, you just lay back and enjoy. The only thing you need to do is put your ankles *toward the sky*."
Synonyms: upward

treasure

"I *treasure* the moments we are lying naked together, or even when we are just all alone."
Synonyms: cherish

"Tonight I am going on a *treasure* hunt, and you are the *treasure*. I don't have a compass, but I know I need to head south."
Synonyms: prize

tremble

"My entire body begins to *tremble* when you tie me up and tickle me."
Synonyms: flutter, quiver

U

unbelievable

"You are an *unbelievable* lover, especially when you _____."
Synonyms: astonishing

under/underneath

"I love to feel your body *underneath* mine."
Synonyms: beneath

undiscovered territory

Exploring new places sexually, like doing something you haven't done before. For example, undiscovered territory may be having sex outdoors or in a place you have both talked about but never tried.
They were entering *undiscovered territory* when they had anal sex for the first time while on vacation at the beach.
Synonyms: unfamiliar, unknown

urge

"The *urge* to kiss you all over is uncontrollable. Can I?"
Synonyms: impulse

V

vacancy

"There's a *vacancy* I need you to fill inside of me."
Synonyms: opening, space

velvet

"Your skin feels like *velvet*, inside and out."
Synonyms: plush, silk

vibrate

"Close your eyes. I want to put something up against your body. The only clue you get is its is going to *vibrate.*"
Synonyms: flutter, shake

vivacious

Doing a few things out of the ordinary can create a *vivacious* lovemaking session.
Synonyms: spirited

vixen

"Every time you wear the color red, it reminds me what a sexy *vixen* you are."
Synonyms: fox

voluptuous

"*Voluptuous* pleasure takes over me whenever you _____."
Synonyms: sensual

voracious

"Whenever you wear those sexy panties or _____ to bed, I get the feeling of a *voracious* appetite for giving you oral sex."
Synonyms: insatiable

voyeur

"Let's role-play where one of us is the *voyeur* and the other undresses and then takes a shower while being watched."
Synonyms: Peeping Tom, scopophiliac

W

wet

"Every time you kiss me on the neck or _____, you make me so *wet*."
"You get so *wet* when we're making love, it makes me even harder."
Synonyms: damp, moist

wet dream

"Good morning, my sweet. I had an amazing *wet dream* with you last night. Let me slip beneath the covers and show you how it started."
Synonyms: nocturnal emission

whiff

"All it takes is a *whiff* of your perfume, and I'm completely aroused."
Synonyms: breath

whisk

"Let me *whisk* you upstairs so I can show you all the things I've been thinking about doing to you all day."
Synonyms: carry, snatch

whisper

They were *whispering* naughty things into each other's ears during the show, and then they went home immediately after to fulfill their plan.

"I'm going to *whisper* into your ear all the naughty things I want us to do tonight."
Synonyms: murmur

wild

"Let's stay in bed all day and have a *wild*, animalistic lovemaking session."
Synonyms: untamed

wonderful

The candle wax play we tried was a *wonderful* experience.
"Your hands all over my ⎯⎯⎯⎯⎯ is such a *wonderful* feeling."
Synonyms: amazing, astonishing, awesome

worship

"Let me *worship* your entire body, starting with your ⎯⎯⎯⎯."
Synonyms: adoration

X

X-rated

"I love when we watch naughty movies together, because soon after, we always get *X-rated!*"

"I love that new move you used last night. It was borderline *X-rated!*"

Synonyms: raunchy

Y

yearn

"They *yearned* for each other over the days they were apart but made up for it as soon as they were together again."
"Watching you eat that strawberry made me *yearn* to kiss your lips."
Synonyms: crave, hunger

yearning

"Baby, I am *yearning* for your lips all over my body, starting with my _____. Then I plan to do the same to you."
Synonyms: desire

youthful

"Having sex in the rain last night made me feel *youthful* again."
Synonyms: young

Z

zealous

"His *zealous* attention to my feet and fresh pedicure, let me know he was into the foot fetish. I'll make sure to tickle him with my toes in all the right places."
Synonyms: enthusiastic

zone (erogenous)

"You know all the right *zones* to touch, kiss, and tickle me to the point where I can't wait to see what will come next."
Synonyms: area, region

Spotlight: Body Part Terms

This section is just to help ensure you have plenty of descriptive words to use when talking about your partner's body or your own. It will help keep you from using the same words over and over and keep bedroom talk fresh and exciting.

breasts. boobs, boobies, bosom, bust, busty, fun bags, gazongas, headlights, knockers, jugs, tits, titties, tatas

butt. ass, behind, booty, bottom, bum, buns, buttocks, derriere, fanny, rear, rear end, rump, tush, tushy, hiney

anus. backdoor, butthole, booty-hole, bum-hole, rear door, rear entry

penis. balls deep, boner, cock, dick, erection, equipment, hard-on, phallus, member, shaft, shlong, tool

vagina. box, cooter, clit, clitoris, cunt, hole, love button, love pit, pink, pink pocket, pussy, vajay-jay

Spotlight: Fetishes

Some people hear the word *fetish* and are immediately turned off or think that fetishes are something unnatural they don't want to explore. This thought generally comes from unfamiliarity with any or all fetishes. It took me a while to understand the differences between the BDSM play practices, and I worked in the industry.

This section is meant to familiarize you and your partner with many of the different types of fetishes to explore and enjoy. They may not all be for you, but you may find one or more that you do want to explore. I like to think that fetishes are just another tool to keep in the tool belt of sexual knowledge. You don't always have to use them, but it's good to know you have the know-how in case you do want to.

Sexual fetishism, or *erotic fetishism*, is the sexual arousal a person receives from a physical object or from a specific situation. The object or situation of interest is called the *fetish*; the person who has a fetish for that object/situation is a *fetishist*. A sexual fetish may be regarded as an enhancing element to a romantic/sexual relationship achieved in ordinary ways. Arousal from a particular body part is classified as partialism.

Bondage. The act of being bound by, or subjected to, some external power or control. The practice of being physically restrained, as by being tied up, chained, or put in handcuffs, for sexual gratification.

Bondage is considered a fetish, as enthusiasts generally prefer the thought or presence of a fully clothed restrained partner to a fully nude and unrestrained partner.

Bondage is not to be confused with the more specific practices of B&D, the practice of restraining and then dominating or humiliating a partner. And it is not to be confused with S&M, the practice of hurting one's partner in order to achieve sexual climax. Bondage enthusiasts generally prefer the more docile forms.

B&D. BDSM is an acronym derived from the term *bondage and discipline* (B&D), *dominance and submission*, (D&S), *sadism and masochism* (S&M).

BDSM includes a wide variety of activities and forms of interpersonal relationships. While not always overtly sexual in nature, the activities and relationships within a BDSM context are almost always eroticized by the participants in some way.

There are many limitless activities incorporated under BDSM, which include sexual role-playing, sexual fetishism, power exchange, dominance and submission, discipline and punishment, sadomasochism, bondage . . .

It is important to know that BDSM is not a form of sexual abuse. Some BDSM activities may appear to be violent or coercive, but such activities are conducted with the consent of all partners involved.

BDSM relationships and practices are exercised under the philosophy of "safe, sane, and consensual" (SSC), or the somewhat more permissive philosophy of "risk-aware consensual kink" (RACK).

Tip: Always use a safe word when engaging in this type of role-play so that if one partner reaches his or her comfort limitations, there is a clear, precise word that conveys to the other partner it is time to stop or slow down and communicate. A safe word can be anything that is not related to the subject of play. The word should be completely nonsexual, such as *Ohio, teapot,* or *Jupiter.*

balloon fetish. A balloon fetish is sexual arousal that involves play with balloons.

Some balloon fetishists revel in the popping of balloons, and others may become anxious and tearful at the thought or act of the balloon popping. Others enjoy blowing up balloons or sitting and lying on them. The origins of the balloon fetish are complex and vary between individuals but may be explained as a form of sexual imprinting.

Many "looners" attribute their fetish to early sexual or presexual experiences with balloons, often involving theirs being burst by members of the desirable sex.

candlewax play. A fetish involving the pouring of candle wax onto your lover's bare body. Start off with areas that are not as sensitive as your private parts, such as chest, back, and buttocks.

Tip: Allow the candles thirty to sixty minutes to burn and build up enough wax. Make sure to hold the candle at least twelve inches from the body to allow the wax cooling time before it hits the skin. You can adjust these tips to personal preference later. Don't forget to lay down a sheet that you don't mind getting ruined if things get really messy.

exhibitionism. (1) A tendency to display one's abilities or to behave in such a way as to attract attention.
(2) A fetish characterized by a compulsion to exhibit the genitals in public or to have sex in public or in a closed environment where other individuals are watching. Examples are a swing party or an orgy.

foot fetish. The admiration or sexual attraction of bare feet. Usually pertains to men who become aroused from the sight of any part of a woman's foot, including soles, arches, or toes. Can also extend to pantyhose, stockings, and high heels. Can be an attraction to painted toes, nonpainted toes, dirty feet, etc. Can incorporate foot jobs, foot worshipping, and toe sucking.

Tip: I highly suggest you and your lover try this out at least once. There are numerous nerve endings in the feet that connect to many pleasure points in the body.

power exchange. A form of BDSM play where partners take turns in both dominant and submissive roles.

S&M. An activity that involves consenting adults using pain as pleasure or a sexual stimulant.

Some practices of S&M include breast/nipple stimulation (nipple clamps), whipping, spanking, tickling, vaginal stimulation, cock and ball torture, bondage, asphyxiation, and hot wax.

sadism. Pleasure is gained from other people's pain. This person would be known as a **sadist**.

sadomasochism. Sexual gratification gained through inflicting pain. One partner inflicts physical/mental suffering on the other, who experiences pleasure from experiencing pain.

masochism. Sexual gratification gained from pain, deprivation, degradation, etc., inflicted or imposed on oneself either as a result of one's own actions or the actions of others, especially the tendency to seek this form of gratification.

spanking. A fetish where consenting adults strike each other on the butt to induce sexual pleasure. Can be done with an open hand, paddle, flogger, whip, or other tool.

Tip: Always use a safe word when engaging in this type of activity.

smoking. A person who has an attraction for someone who smokes. It is most common in men. For men with a smoking fetish, it will amplify any attractiveness a man already has toward a woman if he sees her smoking. Some men are also attracted to more "sweet and innocent" women who happen to smoke.

tickling. A fetish where one becomes aroused by tickling or being tickled. It is also a form of foreplay and can involve bare hands or other simple items such as feathers.

voyeurism. The practice of obtaining sexual gratification by looking at sexual objects or acts, especially secretively. Sexual gratification can be achieved simply by watching others perform sexual acts. Can include masturbating while viewing or not, depending on the person.

worship. Practice of honor or praise toward your partner brings about arousal. Can also be a form of partialism, where worship of a particular body part takes place. Such examples are foot worship, breast worship, or ass worship.

Household Items Transformed into Pleasure Tools

You don't need to run to the local love shop and purchase all kinds of sex toys to explore a fetish or fantasy idea. Many household items can be transformed into pleasure tools. Take a close look around your home for things that might come in handy for your character's role. Here are just a few ideas. Depending how kinky you get, you may just want to think twice before putting that wooden spoon back into the kitchen drawer.

bondage: Men's tie, rope, or a tightly buckled belt.

candle wax: Any household candle. White wax is best, and least messy. Scented or unscented, your choice.

domination/submission: Everything you see on this list! Don't overlook your most basic household item: ice.

foot fetish: Feathers, high heels, panty hose, stockings.

spanking: Wooden spoon, spatula, etc.

worship: What better way to worship your lover's body than with a full body massage? Baby oil, extra virgin olive oil, lotion.

Carnal Knowledge, Fun Sex Facts

These are just some fun, sex-related facts that might encourage you to spend more sexy time with your lover. These are taken directly from the segments I created for my live radio show.

Sleep naked—Sleeping in the nude might not get you more sex, but it will add an element of sensuality to your bedtime routine. Every time you brush up against each other, you will feel soft, smooth skin. Who knows what that can lead to?

Play dress up—Dressing up is not only for Halloween. Does your partner fantasize about a hot fireman coming to the rescue or a sexy nurse giving them a sponge bath? Sharing fantasies, and then finding way to safely act them out, can be lots of fun. If you are worried about you or your partner breaking out in the giggles, don't worry. Laughing together helps couples grow closer. You have nothing to lose and everything to gain.

Flattery—Nothing will make the spark fade quicker than the feeling of being unappreciated. Keep the sexual attraction alive by complimenting each other every day.

Kissing can keep the dentist away—Kissing encourages saliva to wash food from the teeth and lowers the level of acid that causes decay, preventing plaque buildup.

Sex burns calories—77–150 calories per hour for men and 70–120 calories per hour for women.

Warm feet, warm bed—Studies show that when your feet are warm, you are less likely to be cold, even when naked. So there's one good reason to leave the socks on while having sex during those cold winter months. *Best position for sex in the cold weather?* The spoon. You can cuddle under the warm covers and still get frisky. **Tip:** Read a sexy bedtime story together before bedtime to stimulate the mind and get the blood flowing. Or if you are looking to incorporate new positions into your lovemaking, try a Kama Sutra book.

Dance with me baby—Dancing is not only a great cardio workout and great for burning calories. It literally and physically brings you and your partner closer to each other. *Don't know how to dance?* Perfect excuse to learn, and do something fun together. Try learning a sensual dance, such a salsa or tango.

Sex relieves headaches—During the female orgasm, endorphins are released, which are powerful painkillers. So headaches are a bad excuse for no sex. These endorphins are released into the blood stream, producing a sense of euphoria and leaving you with a feeling of well-being. Sex also relieves tension that restricts blood vessels in the brain. *(I know you love hearing this, fellas.)*

Sex to stay beautiful—Scientific studies find that when women make love, they produce amounts of the hormone estrogen, which makes hair shinier and keeps hair smooth. The sweat produced during making love cleanses the pores and makes your skin glow.

Squirting—Female ejaculation that exits from the paraurethral gland, which is in close proximity or part of the G-spot. Liquid should be clear and odorless and is not easily confused with urine.

G-spot fact—The *Gräfenberg spot*, often called the *G-spot*, is defined as a bean-shaped area of the vagina. Some women report that it is an erogenous zone that, when stimulated, can lead to strong sexual arousal, powerful orgasms, and female ejaculation (squirting). The Gräfenberg spot is typically described as being located one to three inches up the front (anterior) vaginal wall, between the vaginal opening and the urethra, and is a sensitive area that may be part of the female prostate.

Anal fact—The physical sensations available during anal sex are uniquely different from vaginal sex. The rectum is lined with nerve endings, some of which signal the brain to "reward" you with pleasurable feelings when stimulated. For a thrusting penis, the ring of the anus can be a new and strong sensation to enjoy. For men, the prostate gland can be a source of powerful pleasure.

Anal Sex Tip: *Always* use a condom when having anal sex, even in a monogamous relationship. The rectum contains lots of infectious bacteria that can cause burning and urethritis of the penis. It is also a lot easier to clean up afterward.

Sexy Spanish Minute

A few fun, sexy phrases that may come in handy next time you meet a hot Spanish-speaking person and want to speak a bit of his or her lingo. These are taken directly from the segments I created for my live radio show.

What's your name?
Espanol—"Como te llamas?" "Cuál es tu nombre?"

Who did you come with?
Espanol—"Con quien venieste?"

Would you like to dance with me?
Espanol—"Quieres bailar conmigo?"

Would you like something to drink? or "Can I buy you a drink?"
Espanol—"Quieres algo para tomar?" "Puedo comprar un traigo/bebida?"

Kiss me.
Espanol—"Besame."

Would you like a ride home?
Espanol—"Quieres que la/lo lleve a casa?" "Quieres te llevo a casa?

Do you have condoms?
Espanol—"Tienes condones?"

***Bonus Phrase** Just for fun and in case of emergency.

Would you like to join the Mile High Club with me?
Espanol—"Quieres ser miembro del Mile High Club conmigo?"

Story Starters

These erotic story starters are much like the fill-in-the-blanks word games we remember playing as kids. The following story starters are something you and your partner can do together to have fun, and they serve as an inspiration to create your own real-life erotic story. They also make great bedtime stories to ignite a little playtime before sleeping—brings a whole new meaning to the phrase *reading a bedtime story.* In bed together and aroused, let the fun begin.

Turn it up a notch. Go live out your sexy story . . .

Phone Call

The other night, the phone rang, and when I answered, I heard the voice of _____. He/She was calling to tell me how much he/she couldn't wait to _____ me so that we could _____. Immediately, I was turned on, because I had never heard him/her talk like that before. The thought of the two of us _____ sent _____ throughout my body. I didn't know what to say, but I knew I needed and wanted to respond, so I blurted out, "_____"

Story Starter 2

Hotel Room

While on the road for a business trip, I got settled into my room, took off my _____, and plopped my tired body onto the bed. I reached for the remote to turn on some TV for a bit, maybe even watch some_____. Before I clicked the remote's power button, I lay in the silence for a moment. Suddenly, from the room next to me, I could hear _____, and I was not sure if my mind was playing tricks on me, so I listened for a moment. And sure enough, I heard two voices caught up in passion. I knew immediately that they were _____, and then I heard the man's voice call out, "_____." The woman replied, "_____!" I had never heard a woman talk like that before—well, except in movies—and it made me feel _____. I began to picture my _____ and me in this hotel room, bodies entangled, shouting out _____ at each other. Completely aroused, I began to _____ myself with one hand. With the other, I reached for my cell phone to call my _____ and . . .

Story Starter 3

Radio Show Caller

While driving home the other night and listening to _____, I came across a sex-talk program. They were talking about _____, something I had never tried but had secretly fantasized about from time to time. As I listened, a caller told a story about a time they had _____ with their lover. *What a(n)_____ experience! I* thought. I so wanted to be that caller on the line sharing such a great sex-perience. I was unsure of how to initiate this talk with my _____, so I decided to write a fantasy letter to him/her. The letter started out by saying how much I fantasized about _____ with my lover and how I hoped he/she would _____ with me. I went into detail about how I wanted to _____ with him/her and how I couldn't wait for _____ . . .

Sex To-Do List Suggestions

"First Ten"

This is the "honey do" list you both will love. Below are just a few ideas to spark your imagination and your sexual appetite. Check off the ones you've already done, and discuss which ones you want to try. On the following pages, create a custom "sex to-do list" with your lover. Set a timeline or goal of when and how you plan to accomplish them. Then you will be ready for a whole new world of sexual adventures.

Sex on the beach. If you have not done it already, this is where you need to start. On the beach, crashing waves, under a star-filled sky . . . Need I say more?

Rent a hotel room for the night. Do all the naughty things you wouldn't dare do in your own home.

Write your own romantic short story. Then go live it out.

Send your lover on a sexy-note scavenger hunt, where sex marks the spot.

Have a one-night stand with your lover. The two of you plan to meet somewhere as strangers. Turn it up a notch and create a "bar name" (a fictitious fantasy name you give to people you meet at a bar or in public).

Join the Mile High Club. Everyone should be a member. Best time is during a night flight. **Tip:** Bring your own blanket. *Caboose Club for trains.

Role-play. Take turns dressing up as each other's favorite fantasy character (e.g., fireman, nurse, and domination).

Skyline sex in Las Vegas. Rent a room on the strip that features a balcony, and after dinner and a show, put on your own private show with the skyline of Vegas as your backdrop.

Skinny-dipping and then having sex in the great outdoors. Turn it up a notch by having sex in the rain.

Motion on the ocean. Get a balcony room on your next cruise. Under the stars, surrounded by only ocean, bathe in nothing but moonlight.

Diamond club (baseball field) or fifty-yard line. This is an especially good one if there is a sports fan in the relationship. Basketball courts and soccer fields are great places too.

"Our Sex To-Do List"

Sex Adventure   Date Completed

1-
Notes:

2-
Notes:

3-
Notes:

4-
Notes:

5-
Notes:

6-
Notes:

7-
Notes:

8-
Notes:

9-
Notes:

10-
Notes:

Who Says You Have to Stop Here? You Were Just Getting Warmed Up . . .

Resources and Reading List

Resources

urbandictionary.com
dictionary.com
relationship.ezinemark.com

Reading List

101 Places to Have Sex before You Die by Marsha Normandy
"Sex positions & Kama Sutra Poses" by *Cosmo* magazine

Dr. Hernando Chaves M.F.T., D.H.S.
Licensed CA Marriage and Family Therapist, Doctor of Human
Sexuality, Clinical Sexologist, Human Sexuality Professor.
www.drhernandochaves.com
@Hernando_Chaves

Chauntelle Anne Tibbals, Ph.D. - *Sociologist*
twitter: @drchauntelle
www.ChauntelleTibbals.com
www.PVVOnline.com

Case Studies and Listeners' Personal Stories

Case Study: Benefits of Dirty Talk for Couples

Numerous experts point out that learning how to talk dirty provides benefits for couples. Some people may not be comfortable talking dirty, but realizing its benefits has caused them to learn how.

One of the main reasons why couples stay together, aside from commitment, is excitement. It's important for couples to increase excitement by having fun and knowing more about their relationship. Learning how to talk dirty can make a relationship more exciting than the usual.

Hearing how they can satisfy each other in bed can make couples more intimate and increase their confidence in having fun. This will make them ask for more from their partners when it comes to lovemaking. Simple things like "I like what you're doing right now" or "Tell me more about your fantasies" somehow open the door to knowing one's partner better and what satisfies him or her in bed. Learning how to talk dirty will make lovemaking more passionate as couples turn their fantasies into reality. Dirty talking can even make them more open with each other.

Countless couples separate, and many of them indicate that they are starting to lose fire when it comes to lovemaking.

This is when they start to feel that lovemaking is just routine and not a passionate moment.

Simultaneously, dirty talking is a good way add some fun variety and help couples interact with each other in bed.

The good thing about knowing how to talk dirty is that it does not require vulgar terms. Being detailed when it comes to asking what you want in bed is enough to consider it dirty talk. Adding a more passionate and seductive tone while saying, "Do it faster," or "Do it again," is enough to improve your skills in talking during lovemaking.

Listener's Story

Glenn had become a regular caller into my radio show. The first time he called he needed advice for an issue that he had been having with his wife for some time.

Like many men, he had the fantasy of being with two women at once. His wife, Sheila, however, wanted nothing to do with it. He wanted to know how he might be able to convince her to do it. He said that it was not about him desiring another woman but about them living out this fantasy together.

I told him that you cannot and should not try to convince anyone to do something they do not want to do sexually, as they may come to regret it and may even resent you for it.

I advised that a safer way to try to indulge this fantasy was to use the scenario as a role-playing experience: while having sex with his wife, the two of them should try having a dialogue about a threesome during intercourse.

"Make it about her," I told him. "Start off with yourself as the spectator, and let her take center stage."

What I meant is to tell Sheila how amazing and sexy she is and how he would love to sit back and watch another woman please *her*.

Ask her to describe in detail what it is she would like this other woman to do to her and how she would want her to do it.

I told him to let Sheila take control of the fantasy scenario and tell him what she would want him to do. Would she want him only to watch, or maybe masturbate?

I talked with Glenn about finding out one of Sheila's fantasies and returning the favor for her. He told me she always had an attraction to firefighters, so I suggested that he become a firefighter for a night for her.

What was it that she liked about them? Did she want to get carried out of danger, or was it the uniform? I advised him to talk to her about it and get enough details to fulfill her desires in a way that was safe and healthy for their relationship.

Everyone has at least one fantasy that they want to experience in life.

Just because you are in a relationship, it doesn't mean you can't live them out, even if your fantasy involves a hot maid giving the full turndown service or a sexy policeman making an arrest with a full frisk.

While it would be unhealthy and potentially devastating to your relationship to go and live these fantasies out with someone other than your partner, there is always a way to find an erotic avenue to satisfy each other's desires, keeping both of you feeling sexually fulfilled.

I advised Glenn to make Sheila's fantasy a reality first, and then she might be more willing to role-play with his.

Glen vowed to follow my advice and call me back with an update the next week.

When Glen called back, he told me that the erotic factor between him and Sheila had gone way up. They had become more open in communicating their fantasies, talking about them during sex, and dirty talking to each other. They were active in living out each other's fantasies one at a time.

He stated that not only had things improved in the bedroom but that the improvement seemed to filter out into the rest of their life. They did more for each other around the house, laughed more, vowed to keep a date night once a week, and felt a spark had been rekindled within their relationship.

Case Study: Dirty Talk via Text/E-Mail

Stacey has been married for a little over three years, and although she loves her husband, she has to be honest: the passion is dying down.

The biggest culprit is the couple's long hours: both work jobs that require long days, and Stacey's husband travels a lot, as he is a truck driver. Exhaustion and distance prevent them from spending time together and being intimate. At the end of the day, while they are getting ahead financially, nobody is really winning.

Stacey knows that she needs to raise the heat in her marriage, but she also knows that if she waits to get things going until Eric gets home, they'll never get it done.

"Eric works on the road and can be away for weeks sometimes," says Stacey. "But he's always on his cell phone or e-mail, so I figured I'd give sending a sexy message a try."

The first time she sent Eric sexy message along the lines of "I can't wait till you get home tonight. I've got something special on," he thought she meant dinner. Clearly, there was an urgent need for action!

With some persistence on Stacey's part, her husband caught on, and their marriage has never been hotter. They are making more time for each other, planning a weeklong getaway to the Bahamas, and even talking about starting a family.

Stacey learned three big lessons she would share with other women.

1. **Just do it**: It might be awkward to get going, but sometimes you just need to take the plunge. If you are nervous or are not sure what your partner would like, start simple. The important thing is to get started and make the connection.

2. **Build anticipation**: Sexy text messages or e-mails enable partners to tease from afar. By reminding a partner of a favorite time together or offering a preview of what you have in store for later, you build the anticipation and create a sense that he can't wait to see you.

3. **Be visually descriptive**: The texts or e-mails can be brief, but they are a great place to focus on one detail, sensation, or idea. Men are visual creatures, and texts or e-mails are a great way to explore that approach.

Listener's Story

The above method is also great for couples just starting out in dirty talk and not comfortable in talking this way face-to-face yet.

This case study reminds me of a listener of my show named Edgar. He called in to ask how to get his wife, Nancy, to talk back to him in the bedroom while having sex.

"She moans and whispers out an, 'Oh, yes,' every now and again, but that's it," Edgar said. "She's very shy."

I advised starting off slow by sending her some sexy text messages throughout the day and getting her to respond that way first. Then I told him he could turn it up a notch and write her sexy notes and leave them somewhere in the house or in her purse. Somewhere only she would find them.

Once she got used to communicating that dialogue through texts or notes as a way to break through her shyness, I told him to try to bring it into the bedroom by telling her how much a particular text or note turned him on and asking her to repeat it as they were making love.

This method is also a great way to stay sexually connected while you are away from your partner for longer periods of time, like while traveling for work.

I asked Edgar to try this with Nancy and to promise to call back and let me know how things went. He agreed.

When Edgar called back a few weeks later, he told me that it took some time to get Nancy to respond with more than giggles. He stayed positive and kept working at it, and slowly but surely she began to respond to him. She then began to feel more confident using this new dialogue, and she even began to send him messages and write him notes on her own.

He knew then that it was time to try my approach of asking her to repeat a phrase from one of the messages that really turned him on.

He said he was not sure how she was going to respond, but he was willing to go for it. He couldn't believe how she immediately responded to him in such a sexy whisper.

Since then, this had become a regular practice in their lovemaking, and the heat factor between them had gotten hotter than ever before. He said things were more erotic then when they first started dating and that the relationship felt brand new again and even more exciting than before.

He thanked me for the idea, and I thanked him for calling into the show and making the effort to make things as good as they can be between him and Nancy.

Author's Note

I am a strong advocate of exploring all the options when it comes to keeping the passion alive within your relationship. After all, you have invested your emotions into this person as well as time that you can never get back.

They say the grass always seems greener on the other side, but oftentimes it is not, once you have gotten there.

If you are happy with your relationship but it needs some fine-tuning, better to invest your time in that than into starting over completely from the beginning in the unknown.

Relationships in my personal opinion are much like flowers or plants. Yes, they should grow naturally, but they always need some nurturing along the way, things like good soil and water and sunlight.

Compromises and making the effort to please your partner are essential, especially if you believe the person is worth it.

-AMR

About the Author

Ann Marie Rios was born in Southern California, in the suburbs of Los Angeles. She entered the sex entertainment and enlightenment industry in 2001. She started out on an Internet radio station, KSEX radio, where for four years she hosted a weekly program focused on sex talk and advice. From that show, she was scouted by Spice TV, where she hosted a live sex-talk and advice show for another four years.

She then moved on to Playboy TV, where she hosted another live sex-talk and advice show for another three years. In 2006, she began hosting a weekly sex-talk and advice radio show on Playboy Radio. Her weekly program ran live for just over three years. In 2011, Playboy Radio launched Playboy Radio Espanol, a Spanish/English "Spanglish" version of Playboy Radio on SiriusXM's channel 569. Playboy Radio then offered her a new show as host of a sex-talk and advice show that airs live every weekday.

Ann Marie has done promo spots on numerous radio stations—not only SiriusXM but also on AM and FM radio stations all over the country and in Canada. She has also done promo spots on Los Angeles radio stations such as Power 106 and guest-hosted on Los Angeles's KDAY 93.5.

She runs her own blog, www.annmariesadventure.com, where she answers sex-advice questions from couples and hopeful singles. She participates in discussion panels with doctors, sexologists, and sociologists. She also hosts live seminars in conventions in major cities, including Los Angeles, Chicago, Miami, and Edison, New Jersey. Ann Marie has also written numerous sex-advice columns for various online magazines, including "Between the Sheets with Ann Marie" on Latina.com, which is also a nationally distributed magazine in the United States. Advice question's or reader's comments can be emailed to Ann Marie directly at annmariesadventure@gmail.com